Carmen Possnig

Training in Space: Resisting Microgravity

AF153192

Carmen Possnig

Training in Space: Resisting Microgravity

Effects of Artificial Gravity Exposure on Orthostatic Tolerance Time

Human Sciences Series

Impressum / Imprint
Bibliografische Information der Deutschen Nationalbibliothek: Die Deutsche Nationalbibliothek verzeichnet diese Publikation in der Deutschen Nationalbibliografie; detaillierte bibliografische Daten sind im Internet über http://dnb.d-nb.de abrufbar.
Alle in diesem Buch genannten Marken und Produktnamen unterliegen warenzeichen-, marken- oder patentrechtlichem Schutz bzw. sind Warenzeichen oder eingetragene Warenzeichen der jeweiligen Inhaber. Die Wiedergabe von Marken, Produktnamen, Gebrauchsnamen, Handelsnamen, Warenbezeichnungen u.s.w. in diesem Werk berechtigt auch ohne besondere Kennzeichnung nicht zu der Annahme, dass solche Namen im Sinne der Warenzeichen- und Markenschutzgesetzgebung als frei zu betrachten wären und daher von jedermann benutzt werden dürften.

Bibliographic information published by the Deutsche Nationalbibliothek: The Deutsche Nationalbibliothek lists this publication in the Deutsche Nationalbibliografie; detailed bibliographic data are available in the Internet at http://dnb.d-nb.de.
Any brand names and product names mentioned in this book are subject to trademark, brand or patent protection and are trademarks or registered trademarks of their respective holders. The use of brand names, product names, common names, trade names, product descriptions etc. even without a particular marking in this work is in no way to be construed to mean that such names may be regarded as unrestricted in respect of trademark and brand protection legislation and could thus be used by anyone.

Coverbild / Cover image: www.ingimage.com

Verlag / Publisher:
AV Akademikerverlag
ist ein Imprint der / is a trademark of
OmniScriptum GmbH & Co. KG
Heinrich-Böcking-Str. 6-8, 66121 Saarbrücken, Deutschland / Germany
Email: info@akademikerverlag.de

Herstellung: siehe letzte Seite /
Printed at: see last page
ISBN: 978-3-639-72380-9

ACKNOWLEDGEMENTS

Firstly, I want to thank my supervisors Prof. Nandu Goswami and Prof. Helmut Hinghofer-Szalkay for all their help and patience and for their enthusiasm in explaining the exciting world of scientific research to me. Secondly I would like to thank Dr. Luis Beck and Dr. Melanie von der Wiesche from DLR, Köln, for inviting me to the DLR and letting me be a part of the research team. Thirdly, I want to thank my parents Eva and Kurt for all their support and motivation and the endless supply of good chocolate. Last but not least, I want to thank Josef Zotter for producing this excellent chocolate and I want to thank the teashop Heissenberger for their wonderful green teas that kept me awake during long nights of writing the following thesis.

Thank you all very much!

TABLE OF CONTENTS

LIST OF ABBREVIATIONS

ADH   Antidiuretic hormone

AG   Artificial gravity

ANP   A-type natriuretic peptide

BMI   Body mass index

BNP   Brain natriuretic peptide

CO   Cardiac output

DLR   Deutsches Zentrum für Luft- und Raumfahrt

ECG   Electrocardiography

EEG   Electroencephalography

ESA   European Space Agency

HDT   Head down tilt

HR   Heart rate

HUT   Head up tilt

ISS   International Space Station

LBNP   Lower body negative pressure

MAP   Mean arterial pressure

NASA   North American Space Agency

NIRS   Near infrared spectroscopy

OTT   Orthostatic tolerance time

PR   Peripheral resistance

RPM   Rotations per minute

SAHC   Short-arm human centrifuge

SV   Stroke volume

TT   Tilt table

LIST OF TABLES

LIST OF FIGURES

1. Abstract in German

Während längerer Raumfahrten gewöhnt sich der Körper eines Astronauten an
Mikrogravitation. Bei anschließender Rückkehr zur Erde ist er plötzlich wieder der
Schwerkraft ausgesetzt. Die Veränderungen im kardiovaskulären System, die dem
Astronauten helfen, um sich in der Mikrogravition zurecht zu finden, führen zurück auf
der Erde oft zum Kreislaufkollaps. Das Hauptziel dieser Studie war es herauszufinden, ob
Training in künstlicher Schwerkraft mit einer Kurzarmzentrifuge die orthostatische
Toleranzzeit erhöht und so Synkopen verzögern kann.

Bei sieben gesunden Männern und fünf gesunden Frauen wurde zwei Mal die
orthostatische Toleranzzeit (OTT) gemessen, vor sowie nach dem Training unter
künstlicher Schwerkraft (AG-Training). Als erstes wurde für 60 Minuten
Mikrogravitation mittels Bettruhe in Kopftieflage simuliert, darauf folgte ein
Zentrifugentraining für 90 Minuten und eine 70.2° Kopfhochlage mit Unterdruck im
Unterkörper, um die individuelle OTT zu erfahren. 28 Tage danach wurde das gleiche
Experiment wiederholt, allerdings ohne Zentrifugentraining. Die beiden OTTs wurden
verglichen um herauszufinden ob Zentrifugentraining (zum Beispiel auf der
Internationalen Raumstation [ISS]) der körperlichen Verfassung von Astronauten
nützlich sein könnte und damit das Auftreten von Kreislaufkollapsen beim
Wiedereintreten in das Erdgravitationsfeld verringert werden könnte.

Die Endergebnisse zeigen eine durchschnittliche Steigerung der OTTs von 2.7
Minuten nach Training unter künstlicher Schwerkraft. Frauen konnten ihre OTTs auf
einen Durchschnittswert von 13.6 Minuten verbessern (durchschnittlicher
Ausgangswert 9.2 Minuten), Männer verbesserten sich von 12.9 Minuten auf 15.6
Minuten durch Training. Die P-Werte der ANOVA Analyse sind 0.0019 (AG-Training
verglichen mit dem Testdurchlauf) und 0.0352 (Vergleich Frauen und Männer).

Wir schlossen daraus dass Zentrifugentraining die orthostatische Toleranzzeit in
Frauen und Männern steigert. Unsere Ergebnisse zeigen dass das Auftreten von
Kollapsen in heimkehrenden Astronauten durch Zentrifugentraining im Weltall
vermindert werden könnte.

2. ABSTRACT

During long-term spaceflights, an astronaut's body adapts to microgravity. Once the astronaut returns to Earth he/she is suddenly exposed to gravity again, and the changes in the cardiovascular system which happened due to the absence of gravity now often lead to syncope. The main aim of this study was to find out *whether an artificial gravity (AG) training using a short-arm human centrifuge would increase the orthostatic tolerance time and consequently delay syncope.*

In seven healthy men and five healthy women, orthostatic tolerance time (OTT) was determined twice, pre- and post-AG exposure. First, microgravity was simulated with a head down tilt for 60 minutes, followed by centrifuge training for about 90 minutes and a 70.2° head up tilt with lower body negative pressure, to ascertain the individual OTT. 28 days later, the same experiment took place, but without the centrifuge training. The two OTTs were then compared in order to find out if centrifuge training (on e.g. the International Space Station [ISS]) would benefit astronauts and diminish the rates of syncope upon returning to gravity.

The resulting times showed an average increase of OTT of 2.7 minutes after AG training. Women improved their OTTs to an average 13.6 minutes (from 9.2 minutes without centrifuge training), while men started with an average of 12.9 minutes OTT, improving it to an average 15.6 minutes after centrifuge training. The P-values resulting from the ANOVA analysis are 0.0019 (when comparing AG training to non AG training) and 0.0352 (when comparing men and women).

We concluded that centrifuge training would increase the orthostatic tolerance time in both men and women. Our results seem to suggest that the occurrence of syncope in returning astronauts could be reduced by performing centrifuge training in space.

3. INTRODUCTION

For thousands of years humans have gazed at the stars, wondering about what they are or even what is beyond. Ever since Yuri Gagarin entered outer space as the first human cosmonaut, circling Earth in 1961, we have come a lot closer to exploring space. Unfortunately, there are things holding us back. While the technology to reach faraway planets seems functioning, our bodies seem to restrain us from leaving. Humans are, of course, adapted to the conditions that Earth provides. On Earth, we have a constant gravity force of 1G - in space, we would be surrounded by microgravity. The human body is adjusted to life on Earth and thus gravity. Our circulation system, our blood pressure regulation system and many more are all dependent on it. Gravity „pulls" our blood downwards to provide an even distribution. Our ancestors started to walk upright more than five million years ago (1, 2). One of the physiological consequences was that in an upright posture, the brain is in a higher position than the heart – thus the regulation of the blood flow becomes even more important, as the heart now has to pump the blood up constantly to ensure that the brain gets enough energy. It makes the human body more susceptible for changes in the blood pressure, a factor that will be significant later. Consequential, we need to find ways to keep our bodily functions up and running, to secure the health of the crew members in a microgravity environment while we aim to boldly go where no man has been before.

3.1. Gravity

Isaac Newton was the first one to describe the nature of gravity back in 1684. He combined Galileo Galilei's work on acceleration, Johannes Kepler's works about planetary movements and Rene Descartes' work about inertia to form his theory about gravitation. He used the Latin word for weight, *gravitas*, to describe the attraction between two masses, known today as gravity. This attraction is particularly strong if the mass of one object is significantly bigger than the other (e.g. Earth versus its moon). Gravity is the force that keeps the moon circulating Earth in its orbit as well as it keeps the Earth in its orbit around the sun. Gravity is thus the force that governs motion throughout the universe.

Earth's gravitational field is stronger than most people imagine – at a height of 400 kilometres above the surface, it is still 88.8% of its strength at the surface. 1G is defined as the acceleration (caused by gravity alone) of an object towards the Earth and is equal to $9.8m/sec^2$. If one drops an apple on Earth, the apple would fall at a speed of 1G. However, if an astronaut in the ISS (at about 400 km height) drops an apple, it seems to float – even though it is falling as well. The illusion of floating arises because they – that is, the ISS, the astronaut and the apple – are all falling together. However they are not falling towards Earth, but rather around it. Due to the fact that all three are falling at the same rate, objects inside the ISS seem to float – they are in a state called zerogravity or microgravity.

To hypothesize that the force of gravity is universal, Newton created a thought experiment (see Figure 1). He imagined placing a cannon on top of a very high mountain. If there was no gravity or air resistance, the cannonball would, once fired into the air, fly in a straight line away from Earth, depending on the direction it was fired. However, if a gravitational force acts on the ball, the path it will follow depends on the velocity with which it was fired. At low speed, it will simply fall back to earth (A). The greater the speed, the farther it will fly before landing (B). If the cannonball gets fired at the proper speed (the orbital speed[1]), it would go on circling around Earth in a circular orbit just like the moon (C). If it was fired even faster than that, the cannonball would go into an elliptical orbit (D) or faster again it would travel off into space and never return (E) (3).

---

[1] The orbital speed of a body (usually a satellite or a planet) is the average velocity with which it orbits the barycenter of a system, usually a body of greater mass. It depends upon the radius of the orbit and the acceleration of gravity in the orbit (3).

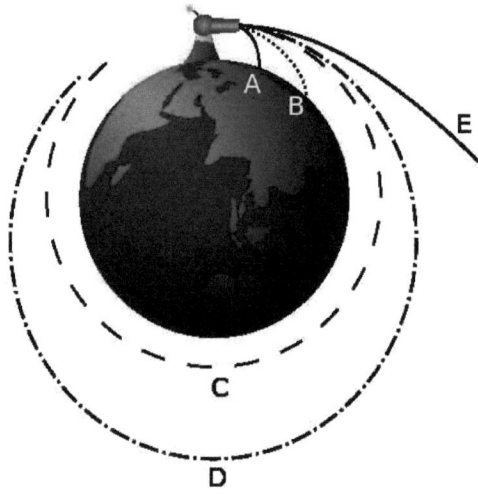

Figure 1: Newton's cannonball. The velocity of the balls rise with A being the slowest and E the fastest. Ball C has orbital speed and circulates Earth like a moon.[2]

For the ISS, or any space ship, the same principle applies. While the apple and the astronaut inside them appear to be motionless and floating, they actually are circulating the Earth at the same speed as the ISS: at 28.000 km/h.

A variety of facilities are used by both ESA and NASA to simulate microgravity. The most known is probably the parabolic flight: an aeroplane flies in a parabolic arc to create microgravity for 20-25 seconds. ESA (as well as the DLR) currently uses the Airbus A300 for parabolic flights, starting in Bordeaux and flying over the Atlantic or Mediterranean. In a predecessor of that plane (NASA's K-135 airplane), the weightless scenes for the movie *Apollo 13* were shot, also in parabolic flight (4).

---

[2] Reproduced from http://m.teachastronomy.com

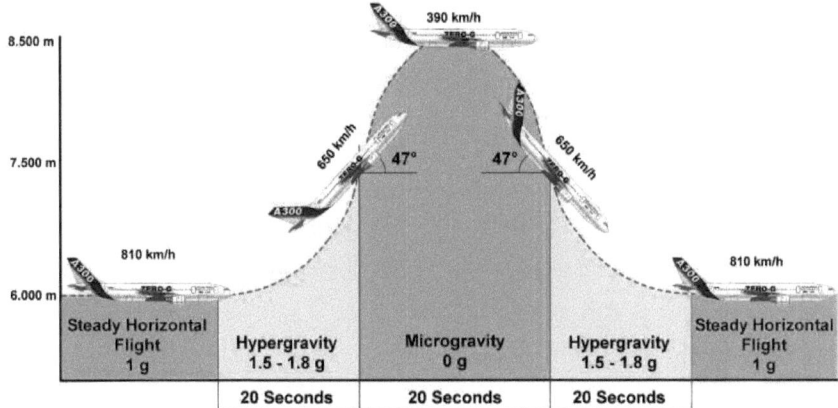

Figure 2: Parabolic flight, entering microgravity for 20-25 seconds[3]

Another facility used to simulate microgravity conditions are drop towers. In the 146 m concrete tower that is situated in Bremen, free falls in vacuum for 4.7 seconds are possible, during which weightlessness can be achieved (5).

3.2. On Earth

3.2.1. Blood pressure regulation

Blood pressure is the pressure exerted by circulating blood on the walls of blood vessels. The pressure varies between a maximum (systolic) and a minimum (diastolic) pressure during each heartbeat. It is principally due to the pumping action of the heart. The mean blood pressure decreases with the distance to the heart getting bigger, resulting in a lower pressure in smaller arteries or arterioles. Most of the fall occurs in the arterioles. Blood pressure is affected by gravity via hydrostatic forces.

As already mentioned, the gravitational force on our home planet is quite constantly 1G. To keep up the blood pressure needed to survive, there are several different mechanisms in our body. Some of them regulate the pressure if there are

_____
[3] Reproduced from http://siliconroadpartners.com/blog/

sudden changes; others are responsible for long-term changes. In addition to these mechanisms, there are many physical factors contributing to the blood pressure. The physical factors can be influenced by various physiological factors, such as exercise, diet, stress, drugs, obesity and diseases. The most important physical factors are fluid volume, viscosity and resistance. The fluid volume affects the cardiac output – the more blood volume there is, the more is transported to the heart – the cardiac output thus increases with the amount of blood circulating. The viscosity or thickness of the blood, which can be changed by certain medical conditions, is important because the blood getting thicker results in a rise of the blood pressure. The relation of resistance to the blood pressure can be described by Poiseuilles' Law. The higher the resistance of the blood vessels, the higher the arterial pressure upstream from the resistance. Resistance is related to

- the vessel length (the longer the vessel, the higher the resistance),
- the radius (the larger the vessel radius the lower the resistance),
- the blood viscosity and
- the smoothness of the vessel walls (the smoothness can be reduced by fatty deposits on the arterial walls).

The size of the blood vessels can be reduced by vasoconstrictors and increased by vasodilators (such as nitro-glycerine). Consequently, vasoconstrictors *increase* blood pressure, while vasodilators *decrease* it. The larger arteries (those who can be seen without magnification) have a low resistance with high flow rates which generate only small drops in pressure, while the small arteries have higher resistance and confer the main drop in blood pressure along the circulatory system.

The blood pressure is a result of the cardiac output and peripheral resistance. An abnormal change in blood pressure is as a result often caused by a problem with the heart's output, the blood vessel's resistance, or both. These connections can be mathematically explained by the following formula:

$$MAP = CO \times PR$$

$$MAP = [HR \times SV] \times PR$$

According to the formula, the mean arterial pressure (MAP) depends on the cardiac output (CO) and the peripheral resistance (PR). The CO is defined by heart rate (HR) multiplied by stroke volume (SV). Therefore, the mean arterial pressure increases if the HR, SV or PR increases, and vice versa. If one of the three terms decreases, one of the others (or both) has to increase in order to ensure a stable blood pressure.

All those interacting factors are regulated by the autonomic nervous system (see Figure 3), and although those individual factors are important, the actual arterial pressure response varies widely because of the short-term and long-term responses of both the nervous system and the end organs.

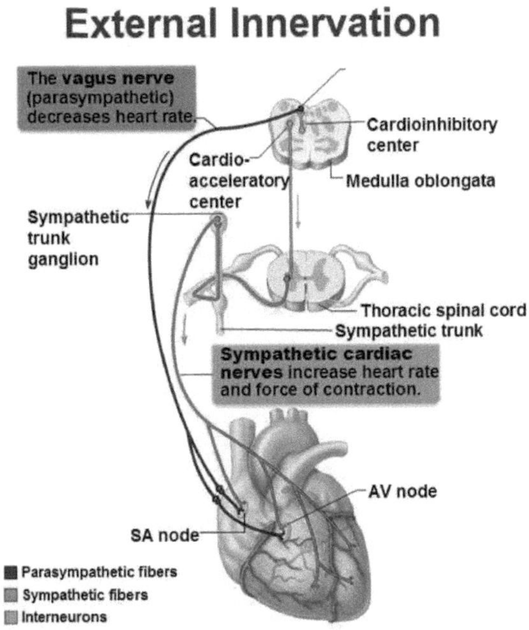

Figure 3: Autonomic regulation of the heart[4]

[4] Reproduced from Tulane University,
http://tmedweb.tulane.edu/tmedwiki/doku.php/intro_to_the_heart_cardiac_electrophysiology

Short-term blood pressure regulation

The short-term blood pressure regulation system consists mainly of neuronal mechanisms, as these are activated more quickly than hormones. For example, if a person needs to suddenly run fast, the sympathetic nervous system will act first and raise the heart rate and subsequently raise the blood pressure as well. Responsible for the most important short term blood pressure regulation are the pressoreceptors/baroreceptors. They are located in the aortic arch and in the carotid sinus (Figure 4). As this is the place where the mean arterial pressure is measured, the baroreceptors give the brain instant information if the pressure changes, thus activating the sympathetic nervous system.

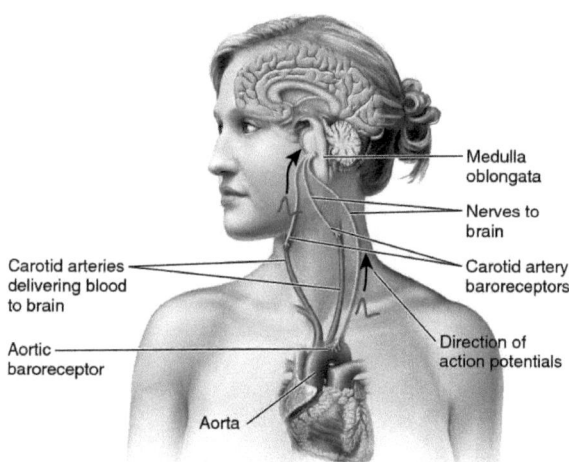

Figure 4: Location of the baroreceptors[5]

The baroreceptors react when there is a sudden change of position, e.g. when one stands up very fast from a lying position. They detect changes in arterial pressure and activate the sympathetic nervous system via the medulla oblongata. The medulla reacts

---

[5] Reproduced from Biology Forums Gallery, http://biology-forums.com/index.php?action=gallery

by altering either the force or the speed of the heart beating, and the total peripheral resistance (6).

Long-term blood pressure regulation

Different mechanisms are responsible for the long-term blood pressure regulation. The adaption of the blood volume to the vessel capacities is the main mechanism. This adaption is reached by controlling the renal elimination of fluids – an increase in blood pressure leads to an increase in renal elimination of fluids and therefore to a decreasing blood volume, consequently lowering the cardiac output. The arterial blood pressure is thus lowered. If the blood pressure should decrease, the reaction runs contrariwise (7).

The renal volume regulation system is conducted by sympathetic renal nerves as well as various humoral factors and hormones. The most important hormonal systems are the renin-angiotensin-aldosterone system, vasopressin, the natriuretic peptides (A-type natriuretic peptide ANP and brain natriuretic peptide BNP) and the kallikrein-kinin-system (6, 8).

The adaption of the blood vessels is conducted by vasomotor reactions and the renin-angiotensin-system: The *vasomotor reactions* are responsible for larger changes in the blood capacity, especially in the splachnicus vessels, while the blood volume is determined by capillary filtration-reabsorption rate as well as by renal fluid elimination in relation to fluid intake. The transcapillary fluid exchange can also help adapt the volume to the capacity, however, this will only permit fluid distribution between intravasal and interstitial volume and is therefore quite limited.

The *hormonal mechanisms* are optimizing the volume regulation. An increased release of renin in the juxtaglomerular apparatus of the kidneys can be triggered by several different events: Every form of reduced perfusion in the kidneys leads to an increase in renin. Decreased intravasal volume will lead to reduced stimulus of atrial receptors and baroreceptors, which in turn augment the activity of sympathetic renal nerves, thus increasing renin release (7, 8).

At low blood volume, the kidneys secrete renin directly into circulation. Renin carries out the conversion of angiotensin to angiotensin I, which is subsequently being converted into angiotensin II. Angiotensin II is a vasoconstrictor and can thus increase the blood pressure, it also stimulates the secretion of aldosterone. Aldosterone has three effects: Firstly, it increases the potassium clearance. Secondly, it increases the reabsorption of sodium and water from the tubules of the kidneys into the blood, thus increasing the blood volume and subsequently the blood pressure, and thirdly, it is a potent vasoconstrictor. At rising pressure, the blood volume is regulated by an increased diuresis. An increased volume in the vessels leads to a lesser secretion of antidiuretic hormone (ADH), which also leads to an increased diuresis (8).

Circulating ANP and BNP block the central effects of angiotensin II, which are ADH release, blood pressure elevation and increased thirst. The natriuretic peptides are thus the antagonists of angiotensin II (8).

The figure below summarizes both the neuronal and hormonal components of blood pressure regulation.

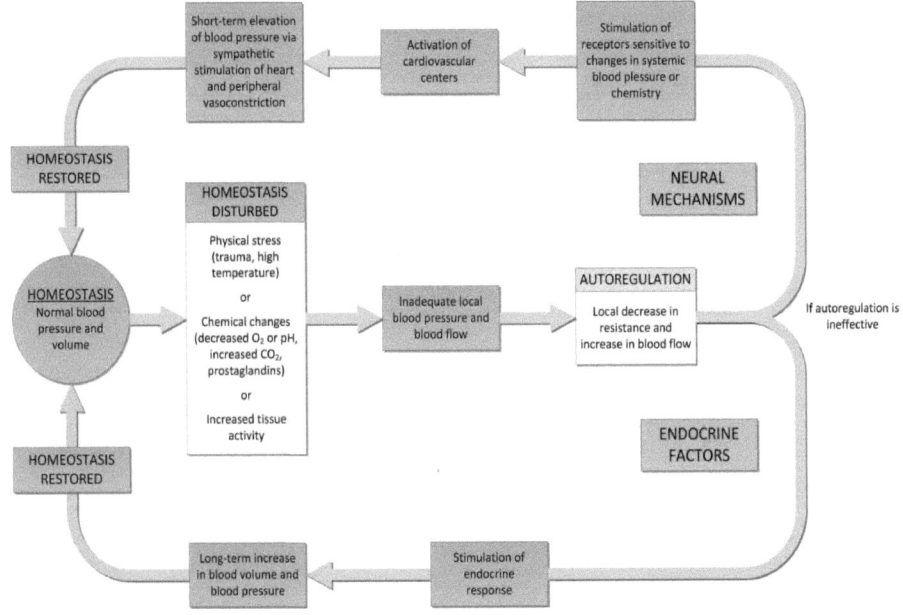

Figure 5: Blood pressure regulation[6]

3.2.2. Orthostasis

Orthostasis is defined as the changing from a lying position to a standing position. It results in a shift of the blood volume and in an activation of circulation controlling mechanisms. During this movement, due to the hydrostatic pressure changes, for a short time there is a 400 to 600ml blood gain in the capacitance vessels of the legs. This blood comes from the intrathoracic vessels, where it is now missing. Due to this the venous return, the central venous pressure, the stroke volume and the systolic blood pressure decrease temporarily (6). To compensate this, the arterial baroreceptors and the stretch receptors in the intrathoracic vessels are activated. The baroreceptors in the aortic arch and in the carotid sinus are especially significant because, while standing, their stimulus

---

[6] Reproduced from http://www.colorado.edu/MCEN/MCEN4278/index_files/Lecture9.pdf

is lower due to the hydrostatic pressure drop, so regulatory reactions are triggered through that as well.

The resistance vessels of the skeletal muscles, the skin, the kidneys and the area around the nervus splachnicus are involved in the vasoconstrictive reaction during orthostasis. In these areas, the blood flow decreases and the peripheral resistance increases (6). The mean arterial pressure reverts to the baseline as a result of the increased total peripheral resistance. Due to the compensatory decline of the vessel capacity, the central venous pressure is only a little reduced. The decreased heart beat volume cannot be compensated fully through elevated heart rate, resulting in the cardiac output being smaller. With some people, these mechanisms do not suffice to keep up a sufficient circulatory support, the blood pressure sinks lower and symptoms such as dizziness, visual illusions or even syncope may occur due to a central inadequate blood supply (6).

3.3.   Going to space

Hypergravity is defined as any force bigger than 1G. Upon leaving Earth on a spaceship, an astronaut's body experiences hypergravity of up to 3G during launch, three times the amount of gravity felt on Earth. The hyper gravity is created by and thus depends on the acceleration force. About nine minutes into the flight, the main engines are cut off. Without acceleration, hyper gravity ceases and the astronauts are immediately under the influence of the microgravity environment. The body can instantly feel the consequences: without gravity "pulling" blood downwards, instead fluids shift upwards into the upper body, increasing the stroke volume (9). It is hypothesized by Norsk et al that the cardiovascular system may even benefit from short-term space flights because of the decrease in the systemic vascular resistance (24+/-4% for at least a week)(10).

3.4.   In space: Human Physiology

When humans enter space, there are a multitude of changes happening to the body, mainly due to the lack of gravity. The human body is adjusted to life on earth. By changing the elemental physics and the surroundings, survival becomes harder.

For humans, outer space is an exceedingly hostile environment. While exploring the universe, our bodies are heavily challenged by the unfamiliar and perilous conditions. The greatest dangers in spaceflight are accidents, a permanent threat in every mission. This is evident from popular incidents such as the 1971 Soyus 11 accident, the fire inside Apollo 1 in 1967, the explosion aboard Challenger in 1986 and the breaking apart of the Columbia in 2003. Since the beginning of human spaceflight some 50 years ago, 18 astronauts/cosmonauts have died in space, and many more in spaceflight related accidents. However, additionally to fatal accidents there are other dangers which endanger an astronaut's health. Firstly, the atmospheric density is reduced as altitude increases. At an altitude of 13km, a pressure mask is needed to breathe; at 20km, the physiological limit for surviving without a spacesuit is reached. And lastly, due to solar flares and cosmic rays from the milky way, the risks of developing cancer, cataracts and damages to the central nervous system (CNS) are elevated (11). And yet, all those dangers combined cannot lessen the curiosity mankind has about space, and the will to explore it. It is possible to minimize the risks an astronaut is taking by entering space, and this study is certainly another big step to ensure that spaceflights to faraway planets such as Mars can be possible without greater health risks.

As mentioned before, gravity affects the distribution of body fluids (Figure 6). While being on Earth, blood is being "pulled" downwards; there is more volume in the lower body (a). Upon leaving Earth's gravity and entering space, this effect disappears and most of the fluids are distributed from the feet, legs and lower trunk to the upper body and the chest (b, c).

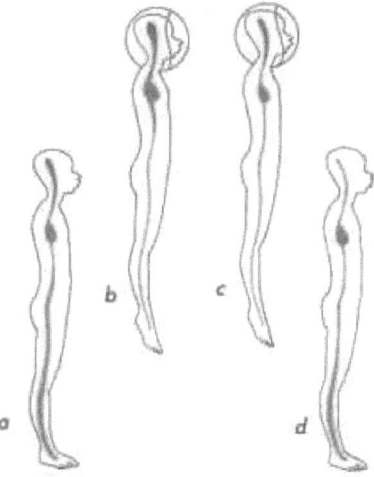

Figure 6: Distribution of body fluids on earth (a), in space (short-term b, and long-term c) and back on earth after spaceflight (d)[7]

As a consequence, at first the heart has to work more and harder to handle the increased volume of blood through the upper body. Even though in total there is still the same amount of blood as before, the receptors in the upper body tell the brain that there is too much. The kidneys now begin to eliminate this "excess" of fluids by increasing the amount of urine - leading to a reduced blood level in the body. This mechanism is followed by another effect of spaceflight: astronauts are less thirsty than on earth, thus reducing the intake of fluids as well, which decreases the amount of blood and electrolytes even more. This volume shift into the upper body causes the "puffy faces" (Figure 7) some astronauts have, as well as the "bird legs" (the legs' circumference gets smaller) (Figure 8) (12, 13).

---

[7] Reproduced from http://www.nsbri.org/HumanPhysSpace/

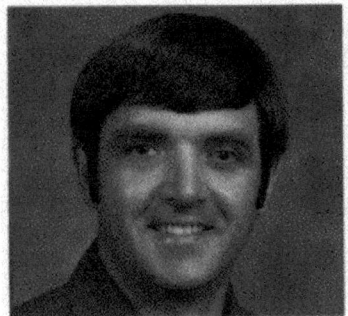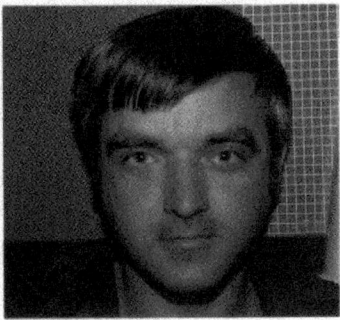

Figure 7: An example of puffy face: an astronaut before (left) and during (right) spaceflight[8]

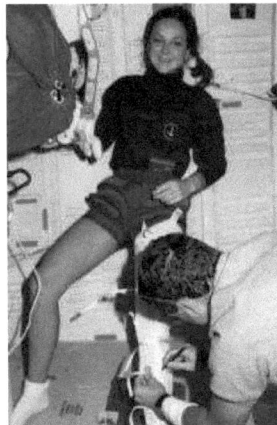

Figure 8: The bird legs syndrome[9]

In the microgravity environment, the heart does not have to work against gravity to get blood into the brain. Additionally, due to the decreased volume of blood circulating, the heart also has less work to do in general. In addition to this, floating around a spaceship takes far less energy than walking on earth. All of this combined may cause the heart after some time to shrink in size (14).

---

[8],[9] Reproduced from http://www.nsbri.org/HumanPhysSpace/

The muscular and skeletal systems are also affected by zero gravity. As they are needed far less in space than on Earth to support the body, they deteriorate over time as the astronauts do not use them. The bones become weaker, loosing calcium, and the muscles atrophy (12). As the bones decrease in mass they loose mineral content and density. There is a typical loss of trabecular and cortical bone volume. The trabecular number and thickness is decreasing, whereas the spacing increases. Additionally, the mechanical strength is altered (Figure 9). The muscles loose mass and volume as well as protein content. There are changes in functional properties and the contractile protein phenotype is altered.

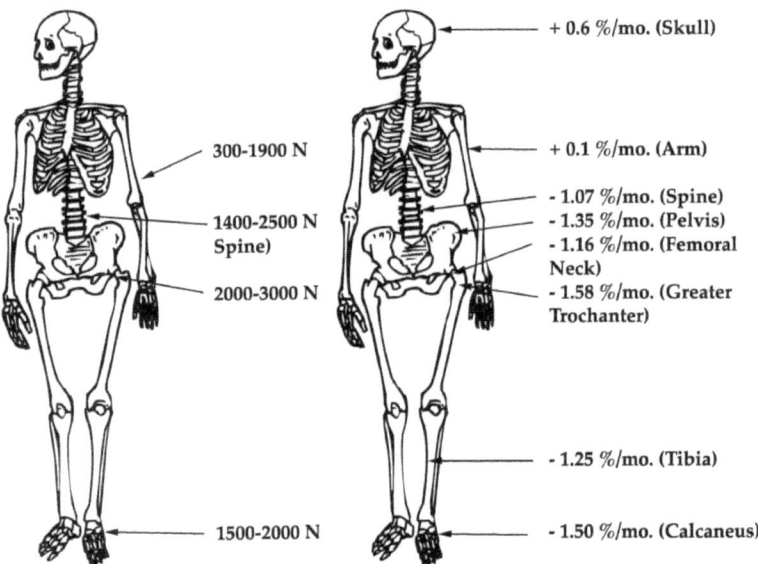

Figure 9: Bone loading on 1G and bone loss in space

Cephalic fluid shifts induced by space flight may lead to increases in cerebrospinal and intraocular fluid pressure, ICP and the loss of visual acuity (15, 16).

Almost all astronauts experience space motion sickness upon entering zero gravity. Usually, the seeing, touching and hearing senses combined give us information where we are, and in what relation to the ground. The vestibular organ in the inner ear is responsible for our balance. It informs the body about movement and spatial orientation, always in relation to gravity. Together with the information from touch, sight and hearing, it enables humans to orientate themselves. In zero gravity, the body is confused, because those senses do not match as they did on earth. Until the body can adapt, many astronauts get sick (this can be compared to sea sickness) (17). The symptoms of space motion sickness can vary from headaches and mild nausea to disorientation and vomiting. For most people, the symptoms last two to four days (12).

Different body functions need different times to adapt to the microgravity environment space provides. As can be seen in Figure 10, each physiological system acclimates at a different rate. The neurovestibular system is the first, causing space motion sickness for the first few days in space, and subsequently adapting to 0G. The fluids and electrolytes are second fastest, resulting in the distribution of the body fluids to the upper body, causing the earlier mentioned "puffy faces" and "bird legs". The cardiovascular system needs considerably more time to adapt to the new environment, followed by the red blood cell mass and the slowly increase in the bone and calcium metabolism. During the time spent in space, there is also a constant slow rise of the radiation effects.

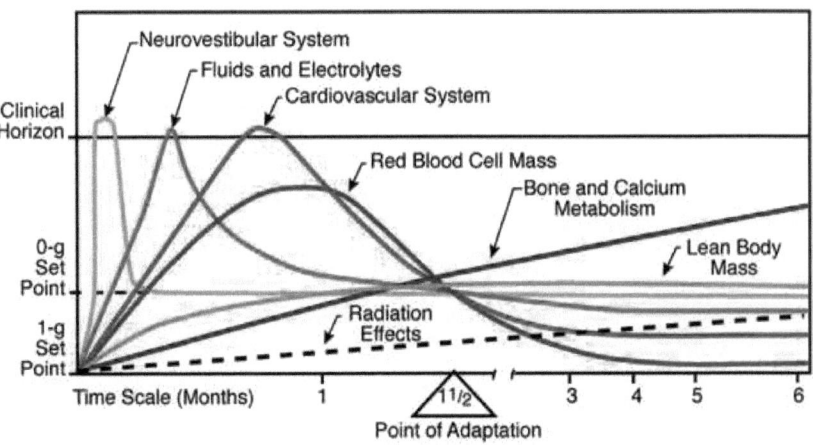

Figure 10: Acclimation to Microgravity

18

3.5.   Returning to Earth

The level of hyper gravity experienced upon re-entry into Earth's atmosphere depends on the speed with which the spaceship approaches. A space shuttle will be under the influence of about 1.2G for 17 minutes, while astronauts inside a Soyuz-Capsule feel the force of up to 7G (or even more) for one minute. Even though it may seem that the G-forces at launch and re-entry are similar, in reality re-entry offers much more difficulties for astronauts, as their bodies are at this point used to microgravity and often have been deconditioned by long flights (18).

3.6.   Back on Earth

Once the astronaut comes back to Earth, gravity takes effect again, pulling the fluids down into the lower body and legs. However, as now there is less blood than before, the upper body and especially the brain will soon lack blood (19). The body cannot compensate this anymore, a situation which often leads to syncope (12). The hypothesis of this study is that the *AG training could delay presyncopal symptoms and thus prolong orthostatic tolerance times.*

3.6.1. Orthostatic intolerance

In most astronauts, the orthostatic instability is proven by elevated heart rate responses to upright posture, but not actual hypotension. After 5 to 16 days of spaceflight, 20% of all returning astronauts during orthostatic challenge experience symptoms severe enough to cause syncope, such as light-headedness, loss of peripheral vision or a sudden drop of systolic blood pressure below 70mmHg (20-25).

Presyncopal astronauts are different from non-presyncopals in their smaller standing norepinephrine levels and their lower total peripheral resistance. In addition, the mean arterial pressure (MAP) is lower (26). The mean arterial pressure is the average blood pressure value; it is independent of the systolic and diastolic up- and downturns. The following formula illuminates the interconnectedness of the single components of blood pressure regulation once more:

$$MAP = CO \times PR$$

$$MAP = [HR \times SV] \times PR$$

The mean arterial pressure accordingly is dependent on the cardiac output (CO) and the peripheral resistance (PR). The CO can be defined by heart rate (HR) multiplied by stroke volume (SV). If either one of the three, the HR, SV or PR, increases, it leads to increases in the mean arterial pressure. The same can be said for the opposite, e.g. if the SV decreases, the MAP decreases likewise, and the HR or PR have to be increased in order to keep the MAP up.

The group of astronauts most likely to be suffering from postflight orthostatic hypotension and presyncope is defined by four major characteristics. The vast majority is female, although not all of them. While all astronauts experience plasma volume loss, those who are presyncopal have less compensatory adjustments. To maintain hemodynamic stability, they are highly dependent on a normal hydration status. Presyncopal astronauts also have low peripheral vascular resistance, before and after flight (26).

3.6.2. Gender differences

Women seem to have greater problems with orthostatic instability after spaceflights. It is not completely understood what the specific mechanisms are; however, they seem to be multifactorial (24). According to a study of 2002 (26), orthostatic hypotension occurring after spaceflights affects mostly women. It is pre-determined mainly by low vascular resistance. After space flight, more women experience presyncope (100% versus 20%). Women also had a greater loss of plasma volume. This is not surprising, as several studies have reported that women have greater risk of getting into orthostatic hypotension than men (27-29). During standing (30, 31), mental stress (32), infusion of pressor agents (33) and cold pressor tests (34), women have greater heart rate responses. In response to lower body negative pressure, standing, mental stress and cold pressor tests, women also have smaller increases in vascular resistances than men (24). Though the single effects are not necessarily a problem,

20

combined with other factors, such as hypovolemia, they can lead to a difficulty to maintain standing pressure.

After the spaceflight, the presyncopal women in the study of 2002 (26) experienced a reduction of plasma volume almost three times greater than the men. In order to maintain an adequate stroke volume, women were very dependent on plasma volume, which put them at an extreme disadvantage. The postspaceflight conditions the women were in induced a collapse of pressure: After spaceflight, the cardiac outputs and stroke volume fell even lower than they had before the flight. Increases in sympathetic responses and vascular resistance did not compensate this (26). These authors suggested that the most important factor explaining the low vascular resistance might be the presence of estrogen. Estrogen has an effect on the endothelium dependent vasodilation: it augments the vasodilation (35-39). This is mediated by nitric oxide (36, 38). The vasodilation consequently lowers the vascular resistance and the venous return.

Another criterion that was put forward by (26) regarding why women are more prone to orthostatic tolerance is the body size. Women are usually smaller and have less muscle mass. However, it has not been proven that more muscle mass affects the orthostatic tolerance in a positive way. The men who did not suffer from presyncope in study reported by (26) had three advantages protecting them from orthostatic hypotension. They have in both supine and standing positions the highest total peripheral resistance. Regardless to plasma volume changes, they maintained their standing stroke volume. And lastly, men produce hyperadrenergic responses to standing on landing day, which is very probably the most important factor, allowing them to increase resistance and maintain pressure (20, 21).

3.7.   Countermeasures of spaceflight induced deconditioning

The exposure to microgravity has direct consequences for humans, some of which are likely to turn into serious medical implications upon returning to earth. Most important are the changes to the cardiovascular and musculoskeletal systems – the fluid shifts and decreased plasma volumes and the atrophy of muscles combined with the negative calcium balance resulting in the loss of bone (40, 41). The body reacts with adaptations to the cardiovascular system, resulting in increased orthostatic deconditioning after returning to Earth. Impaired functions that are experienced post-flight are mainly due to changes in the musculoskeletal system. These changes are mostly evoked by the sudden absence of gravity (11). The countermeasures against spaceflight deconditioning are aimed to prevent those changes as much as possible by simulating Earth-like movements as well as system interactions. One approach to this is exercise (41). Exercise has enabled astronauts to stay relatively healthy during spaceflight missions for well over a year (11). Studies have suggested that very intensive trainings over brief periods may be more effective than low intensity activities (such as bicycling or treadmill training) (41). Although exercise is seen as an effective countermeasure, it cannot prevent significant physiological changes (41). For longer spaceflight missions, such as a mission to Mars, which is estimated to require up to 300 days (in the case of an aborted mission, the astronauts might have to remain in a microgravity environment for up to three years) (40), other countermeasures are needed (11). Artificial Gravity training has shown to improve the orthostatic tolerance time across gender and astronauts practising it in space could be a greatly benefit from it. It is sure to be of great assistance in future space missions, and might facilitate flights to Mars.

Additionally, once astronauts arrive at another planet, they will have to cope with the different environment there. On Mars, the gravitational force is 0.38G. Up to today it is not known whether this would cause deconditioning after landing, as would happen on Earth, or on the other hand if living in a 0.38G environment would be enough to maintain fitness without additional training.

3.7.1. Artificial Gravity

As the name suggests, artificial gravity (AG) is not gravity created by an object or a mass, but is achieved by artificial means. The most important of those means are centrifugal force and linear acceleration. There are two types of AG: continuous and intermittent. Continuous AG can be generated by either spinning the whole spaceship or permanent acceleration at 1G. However, in this study we produced intermittent AG by a short arm human centrifuge (SAHC) and by lower body negative pressure (LBNP).

For long-term spaceflights, generating artificial gravity is particularly desirable. It is proposed that regular AG training can prevent the body getting too used to microgravity and thus prevent the long-term effects of weightlessness on the body. There is a large number of approaches to create AG in space. If mankind is to travel to Mars, Jupiter's moons, Saturn or beyond, we could need more extreme solutions: Such as the early designs of space stations and ships which produce their own gravity: By spinning, rotating around themselves. Several old NASA concepts show giant rotating wheels in space, generating their own gravity by centrifugal force.

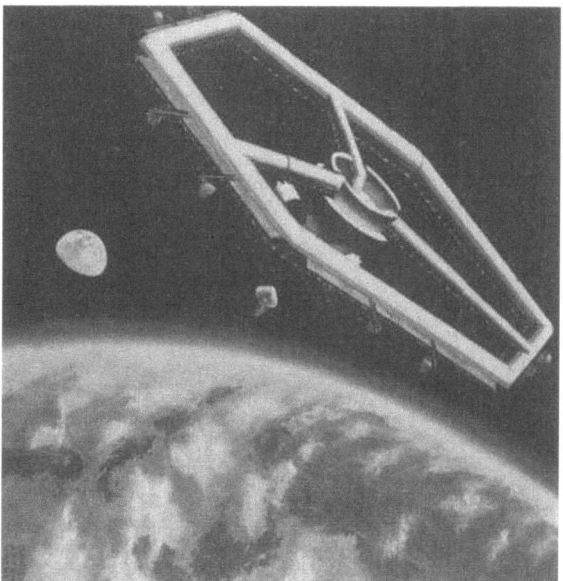

Figure 11: 1962 concept for a manned space station: self-inflating, rotating hexagon, 23m diameter[10]

The artificial gravity effect works thanks to thrusters which rotate the bagel (the wheel) around its axis, generating a centripetal force. Anyone inside this giant wheel will now feel as though they were pulled towards the outer curved hull – although in reality,

[10] Reproduced from http://history.nasa.gov/SP-4308/ch9.htm

it is the floor of the hull which is pushing up against them. Generally, the amount of the artificial gravity produced is dependent on the speed of the rotation and the size of the wheel. The faster the rotation and the bigger the wheel, the greater the effect. In the movie *2001: A Space Odyssey*, this effect is brilliantly shown as the astronaut jogs inside the wheel.

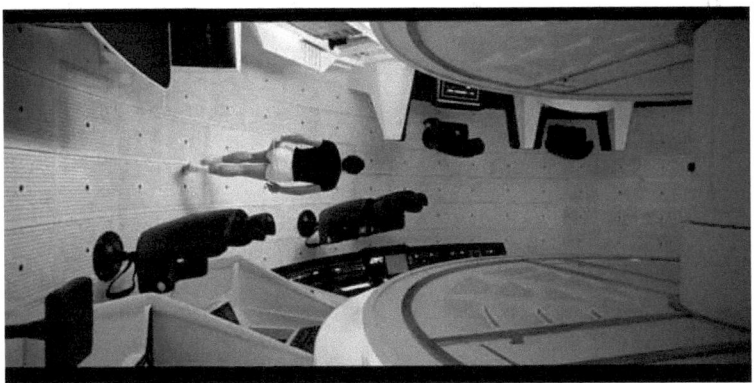

Figure 12: An astronaut jogging in a space ship, scene from 2001: A Space Odyssey[11]

However, a space ship or station like this has not yet been built. As intermittent artificial gravity is much easier and cheaper to achieve, the main focus of this study lies on short-arm human centrifuge training.

3.7.2. Short-Arm Human Centrifuge

With the Short-Arm Human Centrifuge at the DLR, Cologne (www.dlr.de), a test person can be exposed to variable accelerations and G-forces. The main aim for this training is to find countermeasures against the physiological changes due to weightlessness.

---

[11] Reproduced from http://www.centives.net/S/2012/gravity-in-2001-a-space-odyssey/

The maximum acceleration for a lying person is five times the acceleration of gravity. During the SAHC run, the subjects are under constant observation (both medically and technically) with the aid of a control centre outside the centrifuge room.

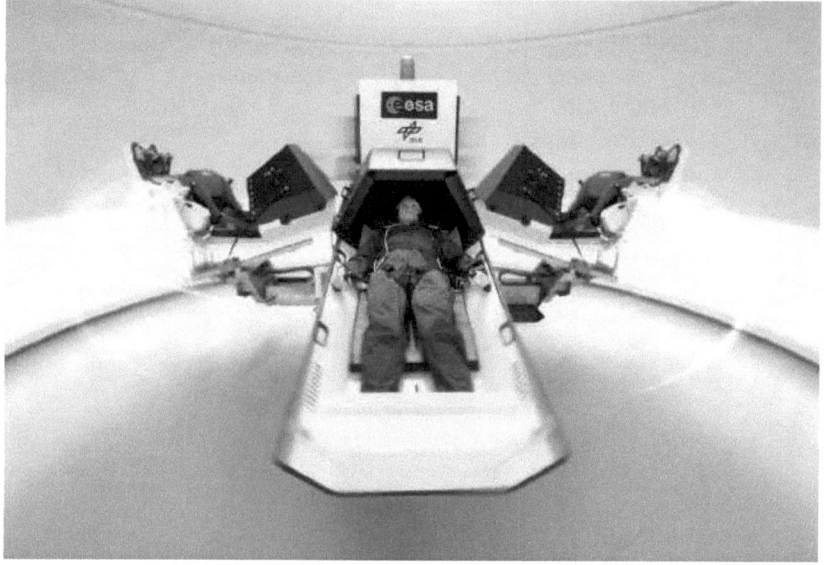

Figure 13: SAHC at the DLR, Cologne

The centrifugal force resulting from the rotation has the following effects on a lying person:

- The skeletal system is being compressed
- There is a shift of body fluids into the lower body and legs
- The semi-circular canals in the inner ear, which are part of the vestibular system and register the rotation movements of the head and body, are being stimulated

It is possible to train a maximum of two probands at once at the DLR's SAHC. They are both stationed at identical positions, either lying or sitting. With both positions, the angle of inclination can be varied, sitting from -10° to +90°, lying to +45°. Additionally, several variations of ergometry are possible.

Human-physiological and technical parameters which can be measured:

- Blood pressure and electrocardiogram
- Spirometry
- Electromyography
- Eye movements
- Oxygen saturation
- Electroencephalogram
- Audio- and video signals

Table 1: Technical data

Max. radius	2.82 m
Max. centrifugal acceleration[i]	~ 5 g
Min. centrifugal acceleration[i]	0.1 g
Max. G- rate of change	~ 0.4 g/s
Max. rotation speed	40 U/min
Min. rotation speed	5.7 U/min
Number and type of gondola	2 beds
	2 seats
Max. bearing capacity	550 kg

- [i] measured at the feet of a lying proband with completely reeled-out centrifugal arm

4. AIMS OF THIS STUDY

The main aim of this study is to test a way to keep the human body in better shape in space. The question is: Can we keep the body used to gravitational forces by applying artificial gravity (AG) training, performed with a short-arm human centrifuge, in space?

In addition, the aim was to find out whether men and women would both benefit in the same way from said training (by delaying syncope), or whether there would be differences across gender. The assumption was that women, being more susceptible to experience syncopal symptoms than men (24), would benefit less from the training than their male counterparts.

In this study the orthostatic tolerance times of men and women were measured and compared. The study consisted of two experiments: the control day and the AG training day. Each of the participants had to attend both days, with a period of 28 days in between the two. This pause was inserted to assure that the women were in the same phase of their menstrual cycle as well as to eliminate any learning effects the centrifugation training might have had. Both control day and AG training day started with a head down tilt (HDT) for 60 minutes. This was done to simulate microgravity since the body experiences similar changes in head down tilt as it does in space: the body fluids relocate themselves in the upper body, especially the brain, and the legs and lower body contain less blood volume. On intervention day, these 60 minutes HDT were followed by the artificial gravity training (with the short-arm human centrifuge, SAHC), which lasted for about 90 minutes, depending on the participant. On the SAHC, the participants were exposed to artificial gravity up to 1.5G. After this they were transferred to the tilt table, where a 70° head up tilt and lower body negative pressure were applied. This simulates the situation when astronauts return to earth's gravity field: The remaining body fluids are being pulled downwards, into the lower body and legs. The upper body as well as the brain suddenly lack blood, the stroke volume decreases and heart is unable to support this situation. The body reacts with syncope. On control day, the protocol was the same save for the AG training which did not take place. As of today, the control day simulates best the situation astronauts are in: first it simulates spaceflight (with the HDT), followed by the return to Earth (by HUT and LBNP). The aim of the study was to find out if AG training with the SAHC benefits the participants and delays the syncope. The aim is to figure out if centrifuge training in space, e.g. on the International Space Station (ISS), would have a benefit on returning astronauts, reducing symptoms of space motion sickness as well as syncopal symptoms when returning back to Earth and gravity. A SAHC on the ISS would simulate gravity in a microgravity environment. *The hypothesis is that this would make it easier for future astronauts to remain healthy during long-time space flights, as well as reduce their affection to syncope afterwards.* We expected their orthostatic tolerance time to increase significantly with AG training. Another question to be answered is *if women would benefit the same way as men from the SAHC training,* or, as they are more prone to suffer from syncope (26), if there is a difference in the change of the OTT.

5. METHODOLOGY

12 healthy Caucasian men and women participated in the study, five of them being female. There were several inclusion, exclusion and drop-out criteria for this study.

Inclusion criteria:

- Healthy female and male participants between 20 and 45 years old, with a BMI between 20 and 26 and a body height between 160 and 188cm
- Non-smoking
- Physically fit, but no competitive athletes
- Successful completion of the medical screening
- Existence of a consent form prior to the experiment

Exclusion criteria:

- Pregnancy
- Smoking, drug or alcohol abuse (more than 20-30g alcohol per day)
- Claustrophobia
- Several diseases, such as
  - Diabetes mellitus
  - Discopathy or eye surgery with laser
  - Rheumatic diseases
  - Cardiovascular diseases or pacemaker
  - Severe orthostatic intolerance or vestibular caused vertigo
  - Kidney diseases (Creatinin >1.20 mg/dl)
  - Anemia (males < 13.5 g/dl Hb, females < 12.0 g/dl Hb)
  - Thyroid diseases
  - Chronic back pain
- Ingestion of drugs which could have influence on the outcome of the experiment
- Any other factor which could have a negative impact on the experiment or the participants' safety.

Drop-out criteria

- Recent illness or disease
- Evidence that the continuation of the study would not be justified
- At any time upon request by the participant

Protocol

Every participant had to be present for two days, the control day (protocol 2) and the intervention SAHC day (protocol 1). Those days were separated by 28 days so that the female participants were in the same phase of their menstrual cycle.

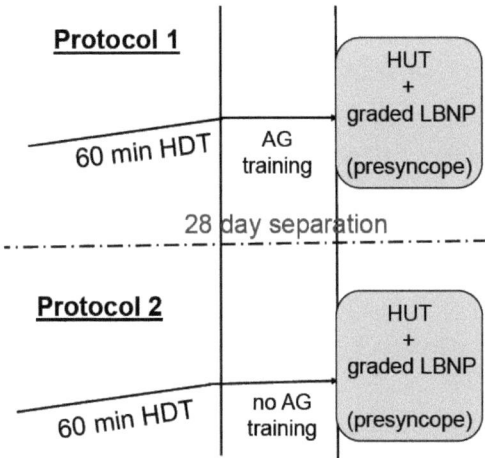

Figure 14: Study procedure

Intervention day (protocol 1) started with a 60 minutes head down tilt followed by artificial gravity training in the SAHC with an adjacent head up tilt and LBNP at the tilting table. Control day (protocol 2) also started with a 60 minutes HDT however no AG training took place. Participants were transported to the HUT and LBNP was applied.

Intervention day protocol:

1. The participant comes to the lab
2. He/she gets instrumented for his/her centrifuge run
3. He/she remains at HDT for 60 minutes
4. Centrifuge run starts
5. The Participant goes through the presyncope determination trial
6. He/she recovers at 0G (5 RPM) for 10 minutes
7. He/she goes through 45 minutes of centrifuge training
8. He/she gets transported to the Tilt Table/ LBNP facility
9. He/she gets instrumented for the Tilt Table
10. He/she gets tilted to 70° head up for 10 minutes
11. LBNP at 20 mmHg is added and held for three minutes
12. LBNP at 30 mmHg is held for three minutes
13. LBNP is increased likewise until presyncopal symptoms appear
14. Return to supine position and 0mmHg LBNP
15. The participant is dismissed by medical monitor

Control day protocol:

1. The participant comes to the lab
2. He/she gets instrumented for his/her head down tilt test
3. He/she remains at HDT for 60 minutes
4. He/she lies still for 90 minutes (equals centrifuge training on intervention day)
5. He/she gets transported to the Tilt Table/ LBNP facility
6. He/she gets instrumented for the Tilt Table
7. He/she gets tilted to 70° head up for 10 minutes
8. LBNP at 20 mmHg is added and held for three minutes
9. LBNP at 30 mmHg is held for three minutes
10. LBNP is increased likewise until presyncopal symptoms appear
11. Return to supine position and 0mmHg LBNP
12. The participant is dismissed by medical monitor

5.1.   Orthostatic Tolerance Testing

Control Day

Experiments were carried out between 8am and 2.30pm. Upon arrival, the
participants were familiarized with the test protocol, they had to return their 24h urine
sample and take a saliva test, as well as a pregnancy test for the females. Monitoring of
blood pressure, EEG, ECG, oxygen and impedance of thoracic region, abdomen and legs
was connected to the participant. Each test started with a 60 minutes head down tilt
(HDT) in the SAHC room, simulating the effects of microgravity and spaceflight.
Participants were instructed to breathe normally and avoid leg movements. After these
60 minutes, participants had to lie supine in a horizontal position for about 90 minutes
(the time they took for AG training on intervention day). They were afterwards
transported in a lying position to the tilt table, where they were lifted 70.2° upwards (as
if standing) for five minutes. After five minutes lower body negative pressure (LBNP)
was applied with a baseline level of -20mmHg, which was increased every three
minutes, -60mmHg being the lowest possible pressure. This simulates the effect of
gravity to astronauts returning from space. The LBNP was stopped and the table tilted to
a horizontal position as soon as the participant experienced pre-syncopal symptoms (e.g.
dizziness, nausea, greyout, paleness, see page 33) or the cardiac output (CO) dropped to
half of the outset value. The time between arriving at 70° head up tilt and the stopping of
the LBNP (at presyncope) is the *orthostatic tolerance time* (OTT). This is shown in the
figure below.

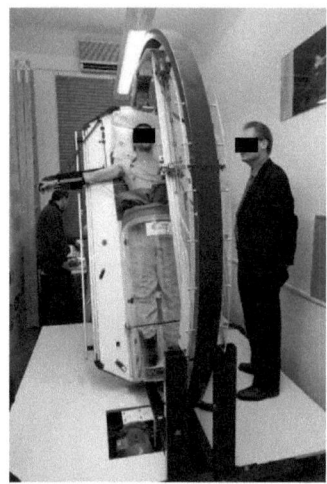

Figure 15: Subject in a head up tilt position undergoing lower body negative pressure.

There were several termination criteria for the Tilt Table testing, at which the Tilt Table was tilted to a horizontal position and the experiment ended.

The termination criteria were the following:

- At any time by request of the participant
- Significant cardiac arrhythmias, such as:
    - Supraventricular or ventricular tachycardia
    - Premature ventricular complexes (repeated or ≥ 6/min)
    - Reconciliation blockades (AV block II or III)
- Haemodynamic criteria, such as:
    - Reduction of the mean arterial pressure < 60 mmHg without increase of heart rate within 60 seconds or reduction of > 40 % of the baseline
    - Heart rate elevation to more than 70 % of the maximal heart rate for more than ten seconds

- Heart rate decrease to less than 50 % of baseline heart rate in the first minute below 50/min lasting more than ten seconds
- Continuous decrease in mean arterial pressure and heart rate lasting more than 15 seconds.

- Clinical criteria, such as:
  - Angina pectoris
  - Slower reaction to speech
  - Nausea, paleness, Vertigo, sweating, paraesthesia

The figure below shows a typical tracing of a subject reaching presyncope. The blood pressure and heart rate of the participant rise constantly during the head up tilt (HUT) and lower body negative pressure (LBNP) phase, until dropping suddenly at LBNP 45.

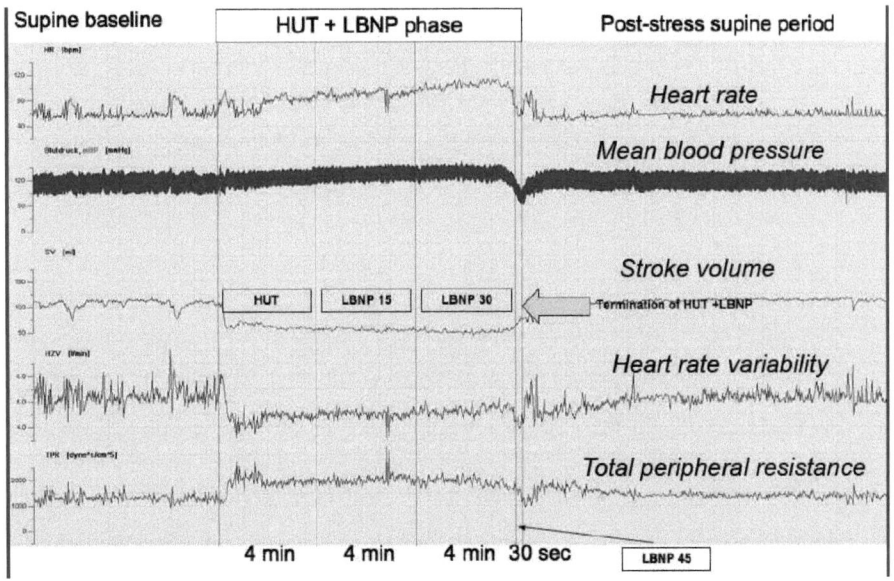

Figure 16: A typical tracing of a subject reaching presyncope

34

5.2.   Artificial Gravity Training

Intervention Day – SAHC

On intervention day, experiments were carried out between 8am and 2.30pm. It started, same as on control day, with a 60min 6° HDT, during which EEG, ECG, NIRS, oxygen, respiration rate, blood pressure, impedance and heart rate were monitored. After this, the SAHC run started, lasting for 75 to 90 minutes depending on the participant. During the SAHC run, the participants were in a horizontal position. They started the centrifuge run with baseline level 0G for ten minutes, followed by ten minutes of 0.6G acceleration for women and 0.8G for men. The acceleration was then increased by 0.1G every three minutes. This continued until the participant experienced pre-syncopal symptoms or the CO dropped to half of the outset value. The participant then returned to baseline level for ten minutes. This presyncopal development test was without interruption followed by two trainings. The first training started at 0.1G lower than the first value of the presyncopal development test, therefore at 0.5G for women and at 0.7G for men for ten minutes. The acceleration was then increased by 0.1G every three minutes until the last level the participant completed successfully in the test run, 0.1G lower than where he had to stop the first time. It was stopped sooner if the participant showed presyncopal symptoms or rapid CO drops. The acceleration was then dropped to the initial value of the first training for ten minutes, and then raised again every three minutes by 0.1G until presyncopal symptoms or rapid CO drops appear. The participant was then transported to the tilt table in a lying position. The tilt table was lifted to 70.2° for five minutes. Following this, LBNP was applied, starting at -20mmHg for three minutes. The LBNP was then raised by -10mmHg every three minutes until the participant showed presyncopal symptoms or rapid CO drops.

The two resulting times were compared afterwards in order to figure out if centrifuge training in space would reduce the symptoms of astronauts coming back to earth.

SAHC Protocol

Presyncope Protocol

Time	G level at heart	
	Female	Male
10 min	5 RPM	5 RPM
10 min	0.6 G	0.8 G
3 min	0.7 G	0.9 G
3 min	0.8 G	1.0 G
3 min	0.9 G	1.1 G
every 3 min	+ 0.1 G until presyncope is reached	

Training Protocol

Time	Female	Male
10 min	0.5 G	0.7 G
3 min	0.6 G	0.8 G
3 min	0.7 G	0.9 G
every 3 min	+ 0.1 G until the level before presyncope was reached, then ramp down to	
10 min	0.5 G	0.7 G
every 3 min	+ 0.1 G until 45 minutes of training are completed or until the level before presyncope was reached	

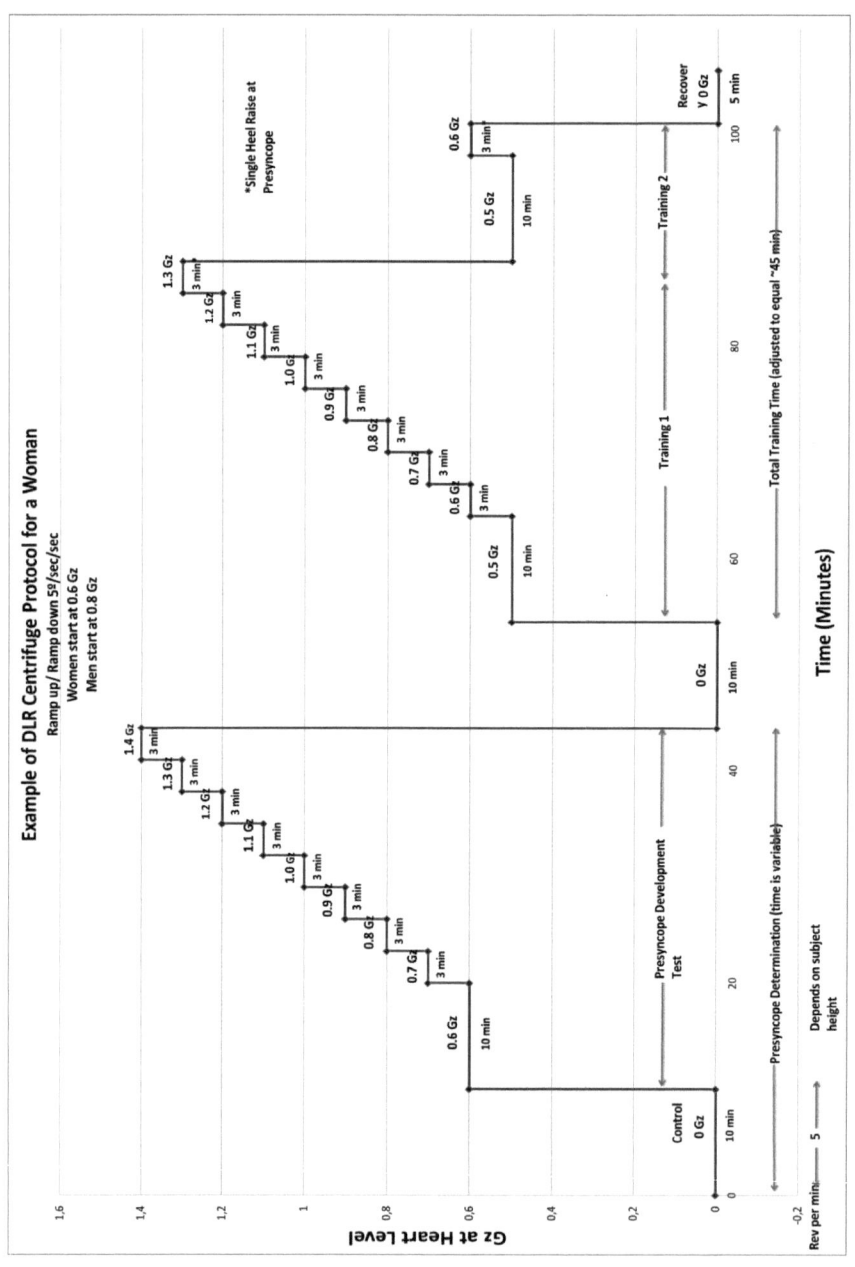

Figure 17: Example of DLR Centrifuge Protocol

6. RESULTS

Twelve healthy Caucasian men and women participated in the study, five of them being female. They were between 20 and 45 years old, had a BMI between 20 and 26 and a body height between 160 and 188cm. All twelve participants reached presyncope using HUT and LBNP.

Table 3 summarizes the orthostatic tolerance time of each participant for the control cay as well as for the AG training day. Participant E was the only one with decreased OTT on intervention day. In average value, participants improved from 11.4 minutes OTT on control day to 14.8 minutes after AG training, showing a significant improvement of orthostatic tolerance time with centrifuge training (Table 6). Looking at men and women separately, it was found that women had an average OTT of 9.2 minutes on control day, which they improved with AG training to an average 13.6 minutes (Table 4). Men had an arithmetic mean of 12.9 minutes OTT on control day, improving to 15.6 minutes after AG training (Table 5).

Table 3: Results (OTT in minutes)

Participant	Sex	Control	AG training
B	M	12.3	15.3
D	M	16.1	16.4
E	M	16.3	15.0
H	M	11.2	12.2
K	F	12.1	17.6
L	F	8.4	10.3
M	M	15.3	17.1
N	F	12.2	15.1
O	M	9.6	16.3
P	F	7.1	15.1
R	M	9.5	17.1
S	F	6.1	10.0
Mean value	F	9.2	13.6
	M	12.9	15.6
	F+M	11.4	14.8

Table 4: Women's OTT results

Participant	Control day	AG training	Improvement
K	12.1	17.6	5.5
L	8.4	10.3	1.9
N	12.2	15.1	2.9
P	7.1	15.1	8.0
S	6.1	10.0	3.9

Table 5: Men's OTT results

Participant	Control day	AG training	Improvement
B	12.3	15.3	3.1
D	16.1	16.4	0.3
E	16.3	15.0	-1.3
H	11.2	12.2	1.1
M	15.3	17.1	1.8
O	9.6	16.3	6.7
R	9.5	17.1	7.6

Table 6: Two-way ANOVA

Table Analyzed Two-way ANOVA	Data 1				
	Ordinary				
Alpha	0.05				
Source of Variation	% of total variation	P value	P value summary	Significant?	
Gender	55.77	0.0352	*	Yes	
Intervention	26.47	0.0019	**	yes	
ANOVA table	SS	DF	MS	F (DFn, DFd)	P value
Gender	150.1	11	13.65	F (11, 11) = 3,140	0.0352
Intervention	71.28	1	71.28	F (1, 11) = 16,40	0.0019
Residual	47.81	11	4.346		
Number of missing values	0				

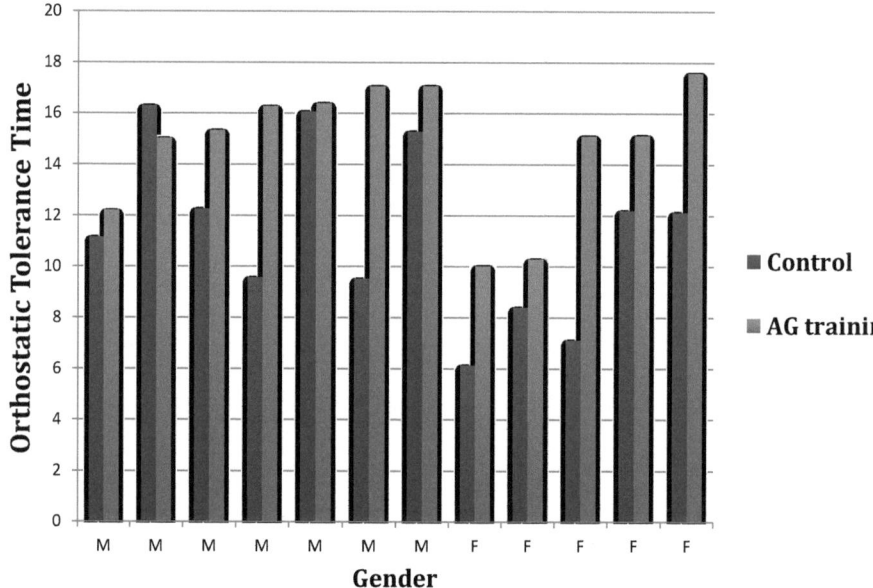

Figure 18: Comparison of Results

7. DISCUSSION

In this study, we investigated if artificial gravity training has a positive effect on the orthostatic tolerance time of men and women. The main aim was to test the hypothesis that short-arm centrifuge training in space would improve the orthostatic tolerance time of men and women, thereby helping to let long-time flights to outer space see the light of day.

Previous studies (42-44) on the subject of centrifugal training have, more or less, always had a similar structure: they discussed and compared the outcomes resulting from different G-trainings. In a 2007 study, Stenger et al (43) demonstrated the usefulness of AG training on improving OTT. Stenger et al tested the OTT of 14 men and 12 women over a three weeks' training procedure. Over these three weeks, every participant was exposed to artificial gravity for 35 minutes a day. The participants were randomly divided into active (performing bicycle ergometry during AG exposure) or passive (no exercise) groups. The experiment took place at NASA's short radius human powered centrifuge. The study had the same training procedure for every participant: a 7min warm-up run at 1G (at the foot), followed by an increase of rotation up to 2.5G for 2min, then returning to 1G. This cycle was repeated during the 35minutes of daily training; however it was not individualized but the same for everyone. The orthostatic tolerance time was determined by a head-up tilt with lower body negative pressure applied, once before and once after the three training weeks. The results showed that men, especially those doing exercise, greatly benefitted from the AG training. The female participants with exercise also benefitted, though less than men, and those without exercise showed no improvement at all. In combination of the active and passive groups, women showed no significant improvement in Stenger et al.'s study. Stenger surmised whether the reason for this is due to the location of the LBNP chamber on the body: the female participants tended to have a larger part of their splachnic region in the chamber. However, as all participants had been given the exact same training, we might speculate a different outcome if participants had their training individualized and tailored to their physical abilities.

Another recent study showed similar results: Fong et al (42) tested six men and five women in a single 60 minutes trial in a short-armed human centrifuge. Again, every participant had the same protocol. They all started at the same level of G-force accelerating the velocity to 2.5G (at the feet), regardless of their individual constitution or whether they are male or female. The 2.5G were then held for 60 minutes. This kind of protocol more than often lead to participants not succeeding in completing the training. If the level of G was too high for them, they would simply stop sooner, thus reducing the training time. The results showed five of six men completing the trial, while in the women's group, four of five trials had to be stopped early because of presyncope.

The striking dichotomy between men and women lead to the exclusion of women from the final experimental protocol. As in the previous study of Stenger et al, Fong et al had the same protocol for every participant regardless of their constitution.

These previous studies have shown that AG training improves OTT in men (43, 44). Their results showed an increase in OTT for men, but little to no effect on women. They concluded that men benefit more from AG training than women do. In general, women seem to have been understudied. Results of previous studies suggest that their tolerance might be lower than that of men, but comparable data are limited. The fact that women often had to stop the training run early lead to each participant having a different length of training period, which of course are difficult to compare among each other.

However, our study showed different results. Our training protocol is significantly different from that of previous studies. The G-training in this study is individualized, matched to each participant's constitution. In our protocol, the AG-training started with a presyncopal development test, determining each participant's level of G tolerance. Afterwards, we trained each person against his or her own presyncope. Every one of the following trainings had an exact time span of 45 minutes. A participant only reaching 1.2G in the presyncopal development test consequently would start their trainings on a lower G level than a participant who reached 1.5G. With individualized training like this, everybody was able reach a training period of 45 minutes, making the results comparable.

Thanks to the individual training, we believe we are the first to report that AG training improves OTT in both men *and* women. Centrifugation has been proven to be a countermeasure to spaceflight induced deconditioning. The two-way ANOVA analysis clearly shows that there is an improvement in OTT for male as well as for female participants after they completed the centrifuge training. The P-value for the centrifuge intervention shows a high significance, with a value of 0.0019. Furthermore this effect has been seen across male and female participants, with a P-value of 0.0352 (Table 6).

On control day, the female participants had a much lower OTT than men (ranging from 6.1 minutes to 12.2 minutes). In average, their OTT was 3.7 minutes less than the men's average. The explanation for this is most probably caused by multiple factors, however the reason is not yet completely understood. Women have a lower vascular resistance than men, and combined with other factors, such as hypovolemia, this could lead to a difficulty of maintaining standing pressure. In addition, women are very dependent on stroke volume to maintain an adequate plasma volume. However, their vascular resistance as well as the venous return are both decreased by the presence of estrogen - as this hormone, with the aid of nitric oxide, augments the endothelium dependent vasodilatation. Another reason for women's lower OTTs could be the body size, as women on an average are smaller than men and have less muscle mass to help pumping blood back to the brain. However, it is not proven that more muscle mass affects OTT in a positive way. In the study of Waters et al (26), the men who did not suffer from syncope had a few considerable advantages: They had the highest total peripheral resistance, they kept their standing stroke volume regardless to plasma volume changes, and they produced hyperadrenergic responses on landing day, allowing them to increase resistance and maintain pressure – probably the most important factor.

However, in our study both men and women showed an increase in OTT. In addition to that, women in general were able to reach higher improvement times. After the centrifuge training women had OTTs ranging from 10.0 minutes to 17.6 minutes. They greatly benefited from AG training, and could increase their OTT by 4.4 minutes (ranging from 1.9 minutes to 7.9 minutes) (Table 4). Across the board men started with higher results (on control day their OTT ranged from 9.5 minutes to 17.0 minutes), and their results after AG training were significantly improved, ranging from 12.2 minutes to 17.1 minutes. Consequently average improvement from control day OTT to centrifuge training Day OTT was 2.7 minutes (ranging from -1.3 minutes to 7.6 minutes). If we ignore participant E, who was the only one decreasing his OTT after AG training, men improved by a arithmetic mean of 3.4 minutes (ranging from 0.3 minutes to 7.6 minutes)(Table 5). Summing up, it appears that women, though having a lower orthostatic tolerance from the beginning, improve more than men – 4.4 minutes for women compared to 2.7 minutes for men. In addition to that, the longest orthostatic tolerance time – 17.6 minutes – was reached by a woman. To figure out why exactly women improve more than men, successive investigations will be needed.

Furthermore, what makes our study special is that each of the participants received a training span which was tailored to their needs regardless of their level of fitness. Through this, we have proved that individualized training is more efficient and has a bigger effect on the individual. This protocol design is completely new to artificial gravity testing and allows the results to be more accurate as it obliterates the personal fitness factors.

Our results are of great importance as microgravity induced deconditioning is one of the most significant problems of human spaceflight. Centrifugation training in space, e.g. on the ISS, could have a positive impact on the constitution of returning astronauts. Performing SAHC training in space would increase their OTT, maybe preventing syncopal symptoms. Further studies will be needed to investigate whether the time span of the AG training could be shortened. We might discover that less than 45 minutes of training would be enough to maintain a good OTT. 30 minutes training, or maybe even 20 or less might be enough. Additional exercise such as bicycle training during the centrifuge run is another promising factor astronauts could benefit from. There is a lot to research, test and discover in the next years and it will certainly bring us closer to exploring strange new worlds.

8. REFERENCES

1. Leakey M,D., Hay R,L. Pliocene footprints in the laetolil beds at laetoli, northern tanzania.

2. Bramble D,M., Lieberman D,E. Endurance running and the evolution of homo.

3. Earth orbit velocity [Internet].; 2012. Available from: http://hyperphysics.phy-astr.gsu.edu/hbase/hph.html.

4. Apollo 13 [Internet].; 2014. Available from: http://www.imdb.com/title/tt0112384/?ref_=tttr_tr_tt.

5. Fallturm Bremen [Internet].; 2013. Available from: http://www.dlr.de/rd/desktopdefault.aspx/tabid-2282/3421_read-5229/.

6. Schmidt L. Anpassung des Kreislaufs an wechselnde Bedingungen. In: Physiologie des Menschen. 30th ed. Springer; 2007. p. 668-71.

7. Busse R. Grundmechanismen der Volumenregulation. In: Schmidt RF, Lang F, editors. Physiologie des Menschen. 30.th ed. ; 2007. p. 665.

8. Busse R. Feinabstimmung der Volumenregulation. In: Schmidt RF, Lang F, editors. Physiologie des Menschen. 30th ed. ; 2007. p. 666-7.

9. Petersen LG, Damgaard M, Petersen JC, Norsk P. Mechanisms of increase in cardiac output during acute weightlessness in humans. J Appl Physiol. 2011 Aug;111(2):407-11.

10. Norsk P, Damgaard M, Petersen L, Gybel M, Pump B, Gabrielsen A, et al. Vasorelaxation in space. Hypertension. 2006 Jan;47(1):69-73.

11. Hawkey A. The importance of exercising in space. Interdiscip Sci Rev. 2003 Jun;28(2):130-8.

12. Lujan B.F. WRJ, editor. Human physiology in space. Houston, TX: National Aeronautics and Space Administration; 1994.

13. Kirsch KA, Baartz FJ, Gunga HC, Rocker L. Fluid shifts into and out of superficial tissues under microgravity and terrestrial conditions. Clin Investig. 1993 Sep;71(9):687-9.

14. Perhonen MA, Franco F, Lane LD, Buckey JC, Blomqvist CG, Zerwekh JE, et al. Cardiac atrophy after bed rest and spaceflight. J Appl Physiol. 2001 Aug;91(2):645-53.

15. Mader TH, Gibson CR, Pass AF, Kramer LA, Lee AG, Fogarty J, et al. Optic disc edema, globe flattening, choroidal folds, and hyperopic shifts observed in astronauts after long-duration space flight. Ophthalmology. 2011 Oct;118(10):2058-69.

16. Polk JD. Flight surgeon perspective: Gaps in human health, performance, and saftey.. 2009.

17. Thornton WE. A rationale for space motion sickness. Aviat Space Environ Med. 2011 Apr;82(4):467-8.

18. Clement G. Fundamentals of space medicine. 2nd ed. Springer; 2011.

19. Goswami N, Batzel JJ, Clement G, Stein TP, Hargens AR, Sharp MK, et al. Maximizing information from space data resources: A case for expanding integration across research disciplines. Eur J Appl Physiol. 2012 Oct 17.

20. Whitson PA, Charles JB, Williams WJ, Cintron NM. Changes in sympathoadrenal response to standing in humans after spaceflight. J Appl Physiol. 1995 Aug;79(2):428-33.

21. Pawelczyk JA, Levine B.D., Neurolab AutonomicTeam. Posturarl regulation of muscle sympathetic nerve activity before and after simulated and actual microgravity deconditioning. Broc First Biennial Space Biomedical Investigators' Workshop League City Texas. 1999:295-6.

22. Buckey JC,Jr, Lane LD, Levine BD, Watenpaugh DE, Wright SJ, Moore WE, et al. Orthostatic intolerance after spaceflight. J Appl Physiol. 1996 Jul;81(1):7-18.

23. Fritsch-Yelle JM, Charles JB, Jones MM, Beightol LA, Eckberg DL. Spaceflight alters autonomic regulation of arterial pressure in humans. J Appl Physiol. 1994 Oct;77(4):1776-83.

24. Fritsch-Yelle JM, Whitson PA, Bondar RL, Brown TE. Subnormal norepinephrine release relates to presyncope in astronauts after spaceflight. J Appl Physiol. 1996;81:2134-41.

25. Meck JV, Reyes CJ, Perez SA, Goldberger AL, Ziegler MG. Marked exacerbation of orthostatic intolerance after long- vs. short-duration spaceflight in veteran astronauts. Psychosom Med. 2001 Nov-Dec;63(6):865-73.

26. Waters W, Ziegler M, Meck J. Postspaceflight orthostatic hypotension occurs mostly in women and is predicetd by low vascular resistance. J Appl Physiol. 2002;92:586-94.

27. Convertino VA. Gender differences in autonomic function associated with blood pressure regulation. Am J Physiol Regulatory Integrative Comp Physiol. 1998;275:R1909-20.

28. Ludwig DA, Convertino VA, Goldwater DJ, Sandler H. Logistic risk model for the unique effect of inherent aerobic capacity on +Gz tolerance before and after stimulated weightlessness. Aviat Space Environ Med. 1987;58:1057-61.

29. White DD, Gotshall RW, Tucker A. Women have lower tolerance to lower body negative pressure than men. J Appl Physiol. 1996;80:1138-43.

30. Gotshall RW, Tsai PF, Frey MA. Gender-based differences in the cardiovascular response to standing. Aviat Space Environ Med. 1991 Sep;62(9 Pt 1):855-9.

31. Schondorf R, Low PA. Gender related differences in the cardiovascular responses to upright tilt in normal subjects. Clin Auton Res. 1992 Jun;2(3):183-7.

32. Collins A, Frankenhaeuser M. Stress responses in male and female engineering students. J Human Stress. 1978 Jun;4(2):43-8.

33. Abdel-Rahman AR, Merrill RH, Wooles WR. Gender-related differences in the baroreceptor reflex control of heart rate in normotensive humans. J Appl Physiol. 1994 Aug;77(2):606-13.

34. Girdler SS, Hinderliter AL, Light KC. Peripheral adrenergic receptor contributions to cardiovascular reactivity: Influence of race and gender. J Psychosom Res. 1993;37:177-93.

35. Lieberman EH, Gerhard MD, Uehata A, Walsh BW, Selwyn AP, Ganz P, et al. Estrogen improves endothelium-dependent, flow-mediated vasodilation in postmenopausal women. Ann Intern Med. 1994 Dec 15;121(12):936-41.

36. Tagawa H, Shimokawa H, Tagawa T, Kuroiwa-Matsumoto M, Hirooka Y, Takeshita A. Short-term estrogen augments both nitric oxide-mediated and non-nitric oxide-mediated endothelium-dependent forearm vasodilation in postmenopausal women. J Cardiovasc Pharmacol. 1997 Oct;30(4):481-8.

37. Arora S, Veves A, Caballaro AE, Smakowski P, LoGerfo FW. Estrogen improves endothelial function. J Vasc Surg. 1998 Jun;27(6):1141,6; discussion 1147.

38. Guetta V, Quyyumi AA, Prasad A, Panza JA, Waclawiw M, Cannon RO,3rd. The role of nitric oxide in coronary vascular effects of estrogen in postmenopausal women. Circulation. 1997 Nov 4;96(9):2795-801.

39. Gilligan DM, Badar DM, Panza JA, Quyyumi AA, Cannon RO,3rd. Effects of estrogen replacement therapy on peripheral vasomotor function in postmenopausal women. Am J Cardiol. 1995 Feb 1;75(4):264-8.

40. Wolfe JW, Rummel JD. Long-term effects of microgravity and possible countermeasures. Adv Space Res. 1992;12(1):281-4.

41. Keller TS, Strauss AM, Szpalski M. Prevention of bone loss and muscle atrophy during manned space flight. Microgravity Q. 1992 Apr;2(2):89-102.

42. Fong KJ, Arya M, Paloski WH. Gender differences in cardiovascular tolerance to short radius centrifugation. J Gravit Physiol. 2007 Jul;14(1):P15-9.

43. Stenger MB, Evans JM, Patwardhan AR, Moore FB, Hinghofer-Szalkay H, Rössler A, et al. Artificial gravity training improves orthostatic tolerance in ambulatory men and women. Acta Astronaut. 2007 0;60(4–7):267-72.

44. Evans JM, Stenger MB, Moore FB, Hinghofer-Szalkay H, Rossler A, Patwardhan AR, et al. Centrifuge training increases presyncopal orthostatic tolerance in ambulatory men. Aviat Space Environ Med. 2004 Oct;75(10):850-8.

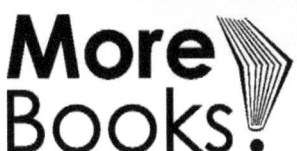
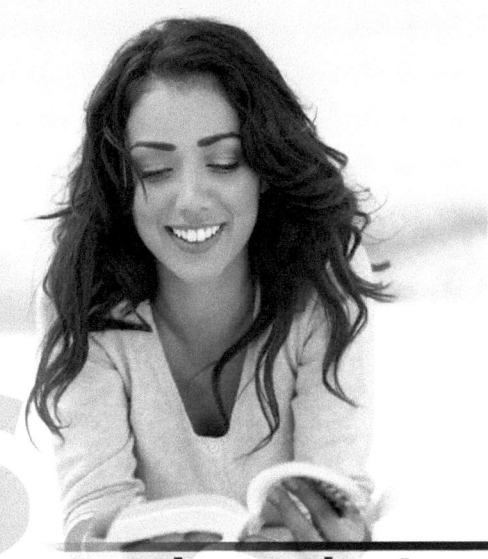
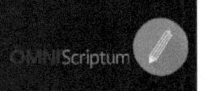

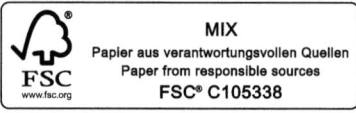

Printed by Books on Demand GmbH, Norderstedt / Germany